THE
GALVESTON
DIET BOOK

Hormone Balancing Revolution for Women Over 40 to Burn Fat, Enhance Diet, Easy and Effortless Way to Lose Weight

MOH LIMS

Copyright © 2023 by Moh Lims

TABLE OF CONTENT

INTRODUCTION

Begin a revolutionary journey with "The Galveston Diet Book," a game-changing technique to effortlessly burning fat and reaching hormonal balance.

This isn't just another welcome; it's a paradigm-shifting guide meant to support you in your weight reduction and hormone-resetting efforts.

As you read through its pages, you'll notice a perfect blend of science and simplicity, providing unrivaled ease in balancing hormonal symptoms.

Discover a wealth of information that will reveal the keys of not just reducing weight but also regaining control over your hormonal well-being.

This book is more than just words; it's a road map to a life in which weight reduction is a natural result of knowing and balancing your body's numerous processes.

Join the numerous others who have embraced this simple yet successful way of life, and let "The Galveston Diet Book" be your guide to long-term weight loss and hormone rejuvenation.

Collagen-Boosting Beauty Smoothie Bowl

Scenario:
Start your day with a delicious and nutritious collagen-boosting smoothie bowl that not only satisfies your taste buds but also enhances your skin's health and beauty.

Packed with ingredients known for promoting collagen production, this beauty bowl is a delightful way to support your overall well-being.

Ingredients:
- 1 cup frozen mixed berries (strawberries, blueberries, raspberries)
- 1 ripe banana
- 1/2 cup Greek yogurt (or dairy-free alternative)
- 1 tablespoon chia seeds
- 1 tablespoon flaxseeds
- 1 scoop collagen powder
- 1/2 cup almond milk (or any preferred milk)
- Toppings: Sliced kiwi, almond slices, and a drizzle of honey

Preparation:

1. **Combine Ingredients:** In a blender, combine the frozen mixed berries, banana, Greek yogurt, chia seeds, flaxseeds, collagen powder, and almond milk.

2. **Blend Until Smooth:** Blend the ingredients until you achieve a smooth and creamy consistency.

3. **Pour into a Bowl:** Pour the smoothie into a bowl, preparing it for the artistic arrangement of toppings.

4. **Top with Goodness:** Arrange sliced kiwi, almond slices, and drizzle honey on top for added flavor and texture.

5. **Enjoy Mindfully:** Take a moment to savor each bite, appreciating the nourishment your body is receiving.

Benefits:

1. **Collagen Production:** Collagen is a crucial protein for skin elasticity and hydration, helping to reduce wrinkles and promote a youthful complexion.

2. **Antioxidant Boost:** Berries are rich in antioxidants that combat free radicals,

protecting your skin from damage caused by environmental factors.

3. **Omega-3 Fatty Acids:** Chia seeds and flaxseeds provide omega-3 fatty acids, which contribute to skin health by reducing inflammation.

4. **Protein Power:** Greek yogurt is an excellent source of protein, supporting the repair and regeneration of skin cells.

5. **Vitamins and Minerals:** Banana and kiwi contribute essential vitamins and minerals, such as vitamin C, which is vital for collagen synthesis.

Application:
- **Breakfast Beauty Ritual:** Incorporate this collagen-boosting beauty bowl into your morning routine for a healthy and beautifying start to the day.

- **Post-Workout Refuel:** Enjoy this smoothie bowl after a workout to replenish your body with essential nutrients, supporting muscle recovery and skin health.

- **Snack with a Purpose:** As an afternoon snack, this collagen-rich bowl not only satisfies your sweet cravings but also nourishes your skin from within.

Remember, while diet plays a role in skin health, other factors such as hydration, sun protection, and overall lifestyle also contribute to a radiant complexion.

Quinoa and Vegetable Stir-Fry with Turmeric-Tahini Sauce

Scenario:

Maintain stable blood sugar levels with a delicious and nutrient-packed quinoa and vegetable stir-fry.

This balanced meal is not only flavorful but also designed to prevent blood sugar spikes, keeping your energy levels steady throughout the day.

Ingredients:

- 1 cup quinoa, rinsed
- 2 cups mixed vegetables (broccoli, bell peppers, snap peas)
- 1 tablespoon olive oil
- 2 cloves garlic, minced
- 1 teaspoon ground turmeric
- 2 tablespoons tahini
- 1 tablespoon low-sodium soy sauce
- 1 tablespoon apple cider vinegar
- Salt and pepper to taste
- Fresh cilantro for garnish

Preparation:

1. **Cook Quinoa:** In a medium saucepan, combine quinoa with 2 cups of water.

Bring to a boil, then reduce heat to low, cover, and simmer for 15-20 minutes or until quinoa is cooked and water is absorbed.

2. **Prepare Vegetables:** While the quinoa is cooking, heat olive oil in a large pan over medium heat. Add minced garlic and sauté for 1-2 minutes until fragrant.

3. **Stir-Fry Vegetables:** Add mixed vegetables to the pan and stir-fry for 5-7 minutes until they are tender-crisp.

4. **Make Turmeric-Tahini Sauce:** In a small bowl, whisk together tahini, soy sauce, apple cider vinegar, and ground turmeric. Adjust the consistency with water if needed.

5. **Combine and Season:** Add the cooked quinoa to the pan with vegetables. Pour the turmeric-tahini sauce over the mixture and toss everything together. Season with salt and pepper to taste.

6. **Garnish and Serve:** Garnish with fresh cilantro and serve immediately.

Benefits:

1. **Stable Blood Sugar Levels:** The combination of quinoa, vegetables, and a balanced sauce helps prevent rapid spikes in blood sugar, promoting sustained energy levels.

2. **Fiber-Rich Quinoa:** Quinoa is a high-fiber grain, supporting digestive health and contributing to blood sugar regulation.

3. **Anti-Inflammatory Turmeric:** Turmeric contains curcumin, known for its anti-inflammatory properties that may help in maintaining overall health.

4. **Healthy Fats from Tahini:** Tahini provides healthy fats that slow down the absorption of sugar into the bloodstream.

5. **Vitamins and Minerals:** The variety of vegetables adds essential vitamins and minerals, contributing to overall well-being.

Application:

- **Lunch or Dinner Option:** Incorporate this stir-fry into your lunch or dinner rotation for a balanced and satisfying meal.

- **Meal Prep:** Prepare a batch for meal prep to have convenient, blood sugar-stabilizing meals throughout the week.

- **Post-Exercise Refuel:** Enjoy this dish after a workout to replenish energy stores without causing a spike in blood sugar levels.

Hormone-Resetting Vegetable Detox Soup

Scenario:

Embark on a nourishing journey with a hormone-resetting vegetable detox soup. This wholesome recipe is designed to provide your body with a variety of nutrients that support hormonal balance and detoxification.

Enjoy a comforting bowl of this soup to reset and revitalize your body.

Ingredients:

- 1 tablespoon olive oil
- 1 onion, diced
- 2 cloves garlic, minced
- 2 carrots, chopped
- 2 celery stalks, sliced
- 1 zucchini, diced
- 1 cup kale, chopped
- 1 cup broccoli florets
- 1 teaspoon turmeric
- 1 teaspoon ground cumin
- 1 teaspoon ground coriander
- 6 cups vegetable broth
- 1 can (15 oz) diced tomatoes, undrained
- Salt and pepper to taste
- Fresh parsley for garnish

Preparation:

1. **Sauté Aromatics:** In a large pot, heat olive oil over medium heat. Add diced onion and minced garlic, sautéing until fragrant and onions are translucent.

2. **Add Vegetables:** Add carrots, celery, zucchini, kale, and broccoli to the pot. Stir and cook for 5-7 minutes until the vegetables begin to soften.

3. **Season the Soup:** Sprinkle turmeric, ground cumin, and ground coriander over the vegetables. Stir well to evenly coat the vegetables with the spices.

4. **Pour in Broth:** Pour in the vegetable broth and add the diced tomatoes with their juices. Bring the soup to a simmer.

5. **Simmer and Season:** Reduce the heat and let the soup simmer for 20-25 minutes until the vegetables are tender. Season with salt and pepper to taste.

6. **Garnish and Serve:** Ladle the soup into bowls, garnish with fresh parsley, and serve hot.

Benefits:
1. **Detoxifying Vegetables:** Cruciferous vegetables like broccoli and kale contain compounds that support liver detoxification, aiding in hormone balance.

2. **Anti-Inflammatory Spices:** Turmeric, cumin, and coriander have anti-inflammatory properties that may help reduce inflammation and support hormonal health.

3. **Hydrating Broth:** The vegetable broth provides hydration and essential minerals, supporting overall well-being.

4. **Nutrient-Rich Zucchini:** Zucchini is low in calories and high in vitamins, contributing to the overall nutrient profile of the soup.

5. **Tomatoes for Lycopene:** Tomatoes contain lycopene, an antioxidant that may have positive effects on hormonal balance.

Application:
- **Hormone-Resetting Cleanse:** Consider incorporating this soup into a short-term cleanse to support hormone resetting and detoxification.

- **Meal Prep Option:** Prepare a batch of this soup for meal prep, providing nourishing and hormone-balancing meals throughout the week.

- **Comforting Dinner:** Enjoy a bowl of this comforting soup for dinner to unwind and support your body's natural detoxification processes.

Fertility-Boosting Quinoa Salad with Avocado and Pomegranate

Scenario:

Embark on a fertility-enhancing journey with a colorful and nutritious quinoa salad. This recipe is carefully crafted to include ingredients known for their fertility-boosting properties, providing a delicious way to support reproductive health.

Incorporate this salad into your diet as part of a fertility-enhancing meal plan.

Ingredients:

- 1 cup quinoa, rinsed
- 2 cups water
- 1 avocado, diced
- 1 cup pomegranate seeds
- 1 cup baby spinach, chopped
- 1/4 cup pumpkin seeds (pepitas)
- 1/4 cup extra-virgin olive oil
- 2 tablespoons balsamic vinegar
- 1 teaspoon honey
- Salt and pepper to taste
- Fresh mint leaves for garnish

Preparation:
1. **Cook Quinoa:** In a saucepan, combine quinoa and water. Bring to a boil, then reduce heat to low, cover, and simmer for 15-20 minutes or until quinoa is cooked and water is absorbed. Allow it to cool.

2. **Assemble Salad:** In a large bowl, combine the cooked quinoa, diced avocado, pomegranate seeds, chopped baby spinach, and pumpkin seeds.

3. **Prepare Dressing:** In a small bowl, whisk together olive oil, balsamic vinegar, honey, salt, and pepper.

4. **Toss and Coat:** Drizzle the dressing over the salad and gently toss to coat the ingredients evenly.

5. **Garnish and Serve:** Garnish with fresh mint leaves and serve the salad chilled.

Benefits:
1. **Folate from Spinach and Avocado:** Folate is essential for reproductive health, and both spinach and avocado are rich sources of this important nutrient.

2. **Pomegranate for Antioxidants:** Pomegranate seeds contain antioxidants

that may help protect reproductive cells from damage.

3. **Quinoa's Complete Protein:** Quinoa is a complete protein, providing all nine essential amino acids crucial for overall health, including reproductive health.

4. **Healthy Fats from Avocado:** Avocado contributes healthy monounsaturated fats, supporting hormone production.

5. **Pumpkin Seeds for Zinc:** Pumpkin seeds are a good source of zinc, a mineral linked to male fertility.

Application:
- **Fertility-Boosting Lunch:** Enjoy this quinoa salad as a wholesome and fertility-enhancing lunch option.

- **Pre-Conception Meal:** Incorporate this salad into your pre-conception meal plan as a delicious way to support reproductive health.

- **Couples' Dinner:** Share this nutrient-packed salad with your partner as a shared meal, fostering a supportive and healthy environment for conception.

Always consult with a healthcare professional for personalized advice on fertility and nutrition.

Alkaline-Boosting Grilled Vegetable Salad

Scenario:

Elevate your well-being with an Alkaline Diet-friendly grilled vegetable salad. This recipe is designed to support hormone balance by incorporating alkaline-forming ingredients that contribute to a more balanced internal pH.

Enjoy this flavorful and nutrient-rich salad as part of your journey towards hormonal harmony.

Ingredients:

- 1 zucchini, sliced
- 1 yellow bell pepper, sliced
- 1 red onion, thinly sliced
- 1 cup cherry tomatoes, halved
- 2 cups arugula
- 1/4 cup extra-virgin olive oil
- 2 tablespoons balsamic vinegar
- 1 teaspoon Dijon mustard
- 1 clove garlic, minced
- Salt and pepper to taste
- Fresh basil leaves for garnish

Preparation:
1. **Preheat Grill:** Preheat a grill or grill pan to medium-high heat.

2. **Grill Vegetables:** Brush zucchini, yellow bell pepper, red onion, and cherry tomatoes with olive oil. Grill the vegetables until they are tender and have distinct grill marks.

3. **Assemble Salad:** In a large bowl, combine the grilled vegetables with arugula.

4. **Prepare Dressing:** In a small bowl, whisk together olive oil, balsamic vinegar, Dijon mustard, minced garlic, salt, and pepper.

5. **Toss and Coat:** Drizzle the dressing over the salad and toss gently to ensure all ingredients are coated.

6. **Garnish and Serve:** Garnish with fresh basil leaves and serve the grilled vegetable salad immediately.

Benefits:
1. **Alkaline-Forming Vegetables:** Zucchini, bell peppers, and tomatoes are

alkaline-forming foods, helping to balance the body's pH.

2. **Nutrient-Rich Arugula:** Arugula is rich in vitamins and minerals, contributing to overall well-being.

3. **Olive Oil's Healthy Fats:** Extra-virgin olive oil provides monounsaturated fats that support hormone production.

4. **Balsamic Vinegar for Flavor:** Balsamic vinegar adds flavor without compromising the alkaline balance.

5. **Anti-Inflammatory Garlic:** Garlic contains anti-inflammatory properties that may contribute to hormonal balance.

Application:
- **Balanced Lunch Option:** Enjoy this grilled vegetable salad as a satisfying and hormone-balancing lunch.

- **Alkaline Dinner Choice:** Serve this salad as a side dish for a well-balanced and alkaline-focused dinner.

- **Post-Workout Meal:** Incorporate this nutrient-packed salad into your post-workout routine for a refreshing and replenishing option.

As with any dietary changes, consult with a healthcare professional or nutritionist for personalized advice, especially if you have underlying health conditions.

Metabolism-Boosting Green Tea Lemonade

Scenario:
Revitalize your metabolism with a refreshing and metabolism-boosting green tea lemonade. This recipe combines the benefits of green tea and lemon to create a hydrating beverage that supports your metabolism.

Make this tea cleanse a part of your routine to kickstart your day or as a pick-me-up during a mid-afternoon slump.

Ingredients:
- 2 green tea bags
- 1 cup hot water
- 1 tablespoon honey (optional)
- Juice of 1 lemon
- Ice cubes
- Fresh mint leaves for garnish

Preparation:
1. **Steep Green Tea:** Place the green tea bags in a cup and pour hot water over them. Allow the tea to steep for 3-5 minutes.

2. **Sweeten (Optional):** If desired, add honey to the hot tea and stir until it dissolves. Adjust sweetness to taste.

3. **Cool and Chill:** Allow the tea to cool to room temperature, then refrigerate until cold.

4. **Add Lemon Juice:** Squeeze the juice of one lemon into the chilled green tea. Stir well to combine.

5. **Serve Over Ice:** Fill glasses with ice cubes and pour the metabolism-boosting green tea lemonade over the ice.

6. **Garnish and Enjoy:** Garnish each glass with fresh mint leaves for an extra burst of flavor. Enjoy your metabolism-boosting tea cleanse!

Benefits:
1. **Green Tea's Thermogenic Properties:** Green tea contains catechins, which may enhance metabolism and promote fat burning.

2. **Lemon's Detoxifying Effect:** Lemon is known for its detoxifying properties and can support digestion, which is linked to metabolism.

3. **Hydration Boost:** Staying hydrated is crucial for maintaining a healthy metabolism, and this tea cleanse provides a delicious way to do so.

4. **Natural Sweetener with Honey:** Honey, if used, adds natural sweetness without the processed sugars found in many commercial beverages.

5. **Vitamin C from Lemon:** Lemon is a rich source of vitamin C, which supports the immune system and overall well-being.

Application:
- **Morning Metabolism Kickstart:** Start your day with a glass of this metabolism-boosting green tea lemonade to wake up your metabolism.

- **Mid-Afternoon Pick-Me-Up:** Combat the mid-afternoon energy slump with a refreshing glass to revitalize your energy levels.

- **Pre-Workout Hydration:** Enjoy this tea cleanse as a hydrating and metabolism-supporting beverage before your workout.

Remember to enjoy this beverage as part of a balanced and varied diet. If you have specific health concerns, it's advisable to consult with a healthcare professional or nutritionist.

Cyclic Hormone-Cycling Smoothie Bowl

Scenario:

Embrace the principles of cyclic hormone cycling with a nourishing and flavorful smoothie bowl. This recipe is designed to align with different phases of the menstrual cycle, providing essential nutrients to support hormonal fluctuations.

Make this smoothie bowl a delicious part of your self-care routine during each phase of your cycle.

Ingredients:

For Follicular Phase:

- 1 cup mixed berries (strawberries, blueberries, raspberries)
- 1/2 banana
- 1/2 cup Greek yogurt
- 1 tablespoon chia seeds
- 1/2 cup almond milk

For Ovulatory Phase:

- 1 cup mango chunks
- 1/2 cup pineapple chunks
- 1/2 avocado
- 1 tablespoon hemp seeds

- 1/2 cup coconut water

For Luteal Phase:
- 1 cup cooked sweet potato (cooled)
- 1/2 pear
- 1/4 cup oats
- 1 tablespoon flaxseeds
- 1/2 cup cashew milk

Menstrual Phase:
- 1 cup spinach
- 1/2 apple
- 1/2 cucumber
- 1 tablespoon pumpkin seeds
- 1/2 cup water or coconut water

Preparation:
1. **Follicular Phase Smoothie Bowl:**
   - Blend mixed berries, banana, Greek yogurt, chia seeds, and almond milk until smooth. Pour into a bowl.

2. **Ovulatory Phase Smoothie Bowl:**
   - Blend mango, pineapple, avocado, hemp seeds, and coconut water. Pour over the first layer.

3. **Luteal Phase Smoothie Bowl:**
   - Blend sweet potato, pear, oats, flaxseeds, and cashew milk. Pour over the second layer.

4. **Menstrual Phase Smoothie Bowl:**
   - Blend spinach, apple, cucumber, pumpkin seeds, and water or coconut water. Pour over the third layer.

5. **Garnish and Enjoy:**
   - Garnish with additional toppings like sliced fruits, nuts, or seeds. Enjoy the cyclic hormone-cycling smoothie bowl mindfully.

Benefits:
1. **Follicular Phase (Days 1-14):**
   - Supports energy and mood with antioxidant-rich berries and hormone-regulating chia seeds.

2. **Ovulatory Phase (Days 15-17):**
   - Provides a boost with tropical fruits and omega-3 fatty acids from hemp seeds.

3. **Luteal Phase (Days 18-28):**
   - A comforting blend with sweet potato for complex carbs and flaxseeds for hormone balance.

4. **Menstrual Phase (Days 1-7):**
   - Hydrating and iron-rich with spinach, cucumber, and pumpkin seeds to support menstrual health.

Application:
- **Cycle Synchronization:** Align this smoothie bowl with the different phases of your menstrual cycle to provide targeted nutritional support.

- **Self-Care Ritual:** Make preparing and enjoying this smoothie bowl a self-care ritual, allowing yourself moments of nourishment and reflection.

- **Share the Experience:** Invite friends or family to join in, making it a shared experience of holistic well-being.

Hormone Harmony Quinoa Bowl

Scenario:
Achieve balance and well-being with a Hormone Harmony Quinoa Bowl, carefully crafted to support hormonal health.

This nourishing and flavorful bowl is designed to provide a mix of nutrients that contribute to hormonal balance, making it a delicious addition to your hormone-friendly diet.

Ingredients:
- 1 cup cooked quinoa
- 4 ounces grilled chicken (or tofu for a plant-based option)
- 1 cup steamed broccoli florets
- 1/2 avocado, sliced
- 1/4 cup pumpkin seeds
- 1/2 cup shredded carrots
- 2 tablespoons tahini dressing (tahini, lemon juice, garlic, salt, and pepper)
- Fresh cilantro for garnish

Preparation:
1. **Prepare Quinoa:** Cook quinoa according to package instructions and set aside.

2. **Grill Chicken or Tofu:** Grill chicken or tofu until fully cooked. Season with your favorite herbs and spices.

3. **Steam Broccoli:** Steam broccoli until tender but still vibrant green.

4. **Assemble the Bowl:**
   - In a bowl, arrange a serving of cooked quinoa as the base.
   - Add grilled chicken or tofu on one side.
   - Place steamed broccoli on the other side.
   - Scatter sliced avocado, shredded carrots, and pumpkin seeds over the bowl.

5. **Drizzle with Tahini Dressing:** In a small bowl, mix tahini, lemon juice, minced garlic, salt, and pepper to create a flavorful dressing. Drizzle it over the bowl.

6. **Garnish and Serve:** Garnish with fresh cilantro for a burst of freshness. Serve your Hormone Harmony Quinoa Bowl immediately.

Benefits:

1. **Quinoa's Hormone-Balancing Nutrients:** Quinoa is rich in essential amino acids, contributing to overall hormone balance.

2. **Lean Protein from Chicken or Tofu:** Provides necessary protein for hormone synthesis and cellular repair.

3. **Cruciferous Benefits from Broccoli:** Broccoli contains compounds that support estrogen metabolism, promoting hormone harmony.

4. **Healthy Fats from Avocado:** Avocado contributes monounsaturated fats, important for hormone production.

5. **Zinc and Omega-3s from Pumpkin Seeds:** Pumpkin seeds provide zinc, essential for hormone regulation, and omega-3 fatty acids.

Application:

- **Balanced Lunch or Dinner:** Enjoy this Hormone Harmony Quinoa Bowl as a satisfying and balanced lunch or dinner option.

- **Meal Prep for the Week:** Prepare components in advance for easy assembly throughout the week, ensuring a consistent and hormone-friendly diet.

- **Post-Workout Nourishment:** This bowl provides a good balance of macronutrients, making it an ideal post-workout meal for muscle recovery and hormonal support.

As with any dietary changes, consult with a healthcare professional or nutritionist for personalized advice, especially if you have underlying health conditions.

Adrenal Support Smoothie Bowl

Scenario:
Recharge your body and support adrenal health with a nourishing Adrenal Support Smoothie Bowl.

This recipe is designed to include ingredients that may help alleviate symptoms of adrenal fatigue and provide a boost of energy. Make this smoothie bowl a part of your adrenal fatigue recovery plan for a delicious and supportive treat.

Ingredients:
- 1 frozen banana
- 1/2 cup frozen berries (blueberries, raspberries)
- 1/2 cup kale, stems removed
- 1/4 cup Greek yogurt (or dairy-free alternative)
- 1 tablespoon chia seeds
- 1 tablespoon almond butter
- 1/2 cup coconut water
- Toppings: Sliced kiwi, granola, and a sprinkle of pumpkin seeds

Preparation:
1. **Blend Smoothie Base:**
   - In a blender, combine the frozen banana, frozen berries, kale, Greek yogurt, chia seeds, almond butter, and coconut water.

   - Blend until smooth and creamy.

2. **Pour into a Bowl:**
   - Pour the smoothie into a bowl, ensuring a thick and spoonable consistency.

3. **Top with Goodness:**
   - Arrange sliced kiwi, granola, and pumpkin seeds on top of the smoothie bowl for added texture and nutrition.

4. **Enjoy Mindfully:**
   - Take a moment to savor each bite, appreciating the nourishment your body is receiving.

Benefits:
1. **Adrenal Support from Berries:** Berries are rich in antioxidants that may help combat oxidative stress associated with adrenal fatigue.

2. **Leafy Greens for Nutrient Density:** Kale provides essential vitamins and minerals, supporting overall well-being during recovery.

3. **Protein and Probiotics from Greek Yogurt:** Greek yogurt contributes protein and probiotics, which are beneficial for gut health.

4. **Chia Seeds for Sustained Energy:** Chia seeds offer omega-3 fatty acids and fiber, providing sustained energy without spiking blood sugar.

5. **Healthy Fats from Almond Butter:** Almond butter adds healthy fats that support satiety and provide a steady source of energy.

Application:
- **Breakfast Revitalization:** Start your day with this Adrenal Support Smoothie Bowl for a nutritious and energizing breakfast.

- **Afternoon Pick-Me-Up:** Enjoy this smoothie bowl as a healthy and satisfying afternoon snack to combat energy slumps.

- **Post-Stress Recovery:** Consume after periods of stress to replenish nutrients and support adrenal recovery.

Remember, adrenal fatigue is a complex condition, and dietary changes are just one aspect of a comprehensive recovery plan. Consult with a healthcare professional for personalized advice and guidance.

Thyroid-Boosting Quinoa Salad with Seared Salmon

Scenario:

Elevate your thyroid health with a flavorful and nutrient-packed Quinoa Salad featuring seared salmon.

This recipe is crafted to include ingredients known for supporting thyroid function, providing a delicious and satisfying dish for those seeking to boost their thyroid health.

Ingredients:

- 1 cup quinoa, rinsed
- 2 cups water
- 1 pound salmon fillets
- 1 tablespoon olive oil
- 1 teaspoon ground cumin
- 1 teaspoon dried thyme
- Salt and pepper to taste
- 1 cup cherry tomatoes, halved
- 1 cucumber, diced
- 1/4 cup red onion, finely chopped
- 2 tablespoons fresh parsley, chopped
- 1/4 cup feta cheese (optional)

For the Lemon-Tahini Dressing:

- 2 tablespoons tahini

- Juice of 1 lemon
- 1 tablespoon olive oil
- 1 clove garlic, minced
- Salt and pepper to taste

Preparation:
1. **Cook Quinoa:**
    - In a saucepan, combine quinoa and water. Bring to a boil, then reduce heat to low, cover, and simmer for 15-20 minutes or until quinoa is cooked and water is absorbed. Allow it to cool.

2. **Seared Salmon:**
    - Pat salmon fillets dry with paper towels. Rub with olive oil, ground cumin, dried thyme, salt, and pepper.

    - In a skillet over medium-high heat, sear salmon for 3-4 minutes per side or until cooked to your liking.

3. **Prepare Salad:**
    - In a large bowl, combine cooled quinoa, cherry tomatoes, cucumber, red onion, and chopped parsley. Add optional feta cheese.

4. **Make Lemon-Tahini Dressing:**
   - In a small bowl, whisk together tahini, lemon juice, olive oil, minced garlic, salt, and pepper.

5. **Assemble and Serve:**
   - Break seared salmon into bite-sized pieces and add to the salad.

   - Drizzle the lemon-tahini dressing over the salad and toss gently to coat.

   - Serve immediately, and enjoy your thyroid-boosting quinoa salad with seared salmon.

Benefits:
1. **Omega-3 Fatty Acids from Salmon:**
   - Salmon is rich in omega-3 fatty acids, which may help reduce inflammation and support thyroid health.

2. **Iodine-Rich Ingredients:**
   - Seafood like salmon and the use of iodized salt contribute essential iodine, crucial for thyroid hormone production.

3. **Quinoa's Nutrient Density:**
   - Quinoa provides a nutrient-rich base with essential vitamins and minerals supporting overall health.

4. **Antioxidant-Rich Vegetables:**
   - Cherry tomatoes, cucumber, and parsley contribute antioxidants, protecting the thyroid from oxidative stress.

Application:
- **Lunch or Dinner Option:**
  - Enjoy this thyroid-boosting quinoa salad as a satisfying and nutrient-dense lunch or dinner.

- **Regular Thyroid Support:**
  - Make this recipe a regular part of your meal rotation to consistently support thyroid health.

- **Meal Prep for Convenience:**
  - Prepare components in advance for easy assembly during busy days, ensuring a thyroid-friendly diet.

Remember to consult with a healthcare professional for personalized advice, especially if you have specific thyroid concerns or conditions.

Balanced Hormone-Regulating Plate

Scenario:

Promote hormonal balance with a delicious and well-rounded Hormone-Regulating Plate. This thoughtfully curated meal includes a variety of nutrient-dense foods known for their ability to support hormonal health.

Make this plate a cornerstone of your balanced diet to foster overall well-being.

Ingredients:

1. **Grilled Salmon:**
   - 1 pound salmon fillets
   - 1 tablespoon olive oil
   - Lemon, salt, and pepper for seasoning

2. **Quinoa and Vegetable Medley:**
   - 1 cup quinoa, rinsed
   - 2 cups water
   - 1 tablespoon olive oil
   - 1 bell pepper (any color), diced
   - 1 zucchini, sliced
   - 1 cup cherry tomatoes, halved
   - 2 cloves garlic, minced

- Salt, pepper, and herbs (rosemary, thyme) for seasoning

3. **Leafy Greens Salad:**
   - 2 cups mixed leafy greens (kale, spinach, arugula)
   - 1/2 avocado, sliced
   - 1/4 cup walnuts, chopped
   - 1 tablespoon balsamic vinaigrette dressing

Preparation:
1. **Grilled Salmon:**
   - Preheat the grill. Rub salmon fillets with olive oil, season with lemon, salt, and pepper.

   - Grill for 3-4 minutes per side or until cooked to your liking.

2. **Quinoa and Vegetable Medley:**
   - In a saucepan, combine quinoa and water. Bring to a boil, then simmer for 15-20 minutes until quinoa is cooked.

   - In a separate pan, sauté bell pepper, zucchini, cherry tomatoes, and minced garlic in olive oil.

Season with salt, pepper, and herbs.

- Mix the cooked quinoa with the sautéed vegetables.

3. **Leafy Greens Salad:**
   - Toss mixed greens with avocado slices and chopped walnuts.

   - Drizzle with balsamic vinaigrette dressing and toss gently.

4. **Assemble the Plate:**
   - Place a portion of the quinoa and vegetable medley on the plate.

   - Add the grilled salmon fillet beside the quinoa.

   - Serve the leafy greens salad on the side.

Benefits:
1. **Omega-3 Fatty Acids from Salmon:**
   - Supports hormone production and regulation.

2. **Fiber and Nutrients from Quinoa and Vegetables:**
   - Aids digestion and provides essential vitamins and minerals.

3. **Healthy Fats from Avocado and Walnuts:**
   - Contributes to hormonal balance and overall well-being.

4. **Leafy Greens for Detoxification:**
   - Supports liver function and helps eliminate excess hormones.

Application:
- **Balanced Dinner Option:**
  - Enjoy this Hormone-Regulating Plate as a nutritious and satisfying dinner.

- **Regular Hormonal Support:**
  - Make this recipe a regular part of your meal rotation to consistently support hormonal health.

- **Post-Exercise Nourishment:**
  - Consume after a workout to replenish energy stores and support hormone balance.

Remember to consult with a healthcare professional for personalized advice, especially if you have specific hormonal concerns or conditions.

Omega-3 Rich Baked Salmon with Turmeric and Ginger Quinoa

Scenario:

Embrace the power of an anti-inflammatory Omega-3 diet with a flavorful and nutrient-packed meal.

This recipe features baked salmon, rich in omega-3 fatty acids, paired with turmeric and ginger-infused quinoa. It's a delicious and health-promoting dish to support overall well-being.

Ingredients:

For Baked Salmon:
- 1 pound salmon fillets
- 2 tablespoons olive oil
- 1 teaspoon smoked paprika
- 1 teaspoon garlic powder
- Salt and pepper to taste
- Lemon wedges for serving

For Turmeric and Ginger Quinoa:
- 1 cup quinoa, rinsed
- 2 cups water
- 1 tablespoon olive oil
- 1 teaspoon ground turmeric

- 1 teaspoon fresh ginger, grated
- Salt and pepper to taste
- Fresh cilantro for garnish

Preparation:
1. **Baked Salmon:**
   - Preheat the oven to 400°F (200°C).

   - Place salmon fillets on a baking sheet lined with parchment paper.

   - Drizzle olive oil over the salmon and season with smoked paprika, garlic powder, salt, and pepper.

   - Bake for 12-15 minutes or until the salmon is cooked through and flakes easily. Serve with lemon wedges.

2. **Turmeric and Ginger Quinoa:**
   - In a saucepan, combine quinoa and water. Bring to a boil, then reduce heat to low, cover, and simmer for 15-20 minutes or until quinoa is cooked.

   - In a separate pan, heat olive oil over medium heat. Add ground turmeric, grated ginger, salt, and

pepper. Sauté for 1-2 minutes until fragrant.
- Mix the turmeric and ginger mixture into the cooked quinoa. Fluff the quinoa with a fork.
- Garnish with fresh cilantro before serving.

Benefits:
1. **Omega-3 Fatty Acids from Salmon:**
   - Supports heart health, reduces inflammation, and may benefit brain function.

2. **Anti-Inflammatory Turmeric:**
   - Curcumin, the active compound in turmeric, has potent anti-inflammatory properties.

3. **Ginger for Digestive Health:**
   - Ginger contains bioactive compounds with anti-inflammatory and antioxidant effects.

4. **Quinoa's Nutrient Density:**
   - A good source of protein, fiber, and various vitamins and minerals.

Application:

- **Balanced Dinner Option:**
  - Enjoy this Omega-3 rich meal as a delicious and satisfying dinner.

- **Regular Anti-Inflammatory Support:**
  - Make this recipe a regular part of your meal rotation to consistently support anti-inflammatory efforts.

- **Post-Workout Recovery:**
  - Consume after exercise to provide essential nutrients for recovery and inflammation reduction.

As with any dietary changes, consult with a healthcare professional or nutritionist for personalized advice, especially if you have specific health concerns or conditions.

Hormone-Boosting Detox Salad with Lemon-Tahini Dressing

Scenario:

Revitalize your body and support hormone balance with a nourishing Hormone-Boosting Detox Salad.

This recipe combines detoxifying vegetables, hormone-supporting ingredients, and a zesty lemon-tahini dressing to create a delicious and cleansing meal. Make this salad a key element of your hormone-boosting detox routine.

Ingredients:

For the Salad:

- 4 cups mixed leafy greens (kale, spinach, arugula)
- 1 cucumber, thinly sliced
- 1 cup broccoli florets, blanched
- 1 cup cherry tomatoes, halved
- 1/2 red onion, thinly sliced
- 1/4 cup pumpkin seeds
- 1/4 cup dried cranberries (unsweetened)

For the Lemon-Tahini Dressing:

- 2 tablespoons tahini
- Juice of 1 lemon

- 2 tablespoons extra-virgin olive oil
- 1 clove garlic, minced
- Salt and pepper to taste
- Water (as needed to thin the dressing)

Preparation:
1. **Prepare the Salad:**
   - In a large bowl, combine the mixed leafy greens, cucumber slices, blanched broccoli florets, cherry tomatoes, red onion slices, pumpkin seeds, and dried cranberries.

2. **Make the Lemon-Tahini Dressing:**
   - In a small bowl, whisk together tahini, lemon juice, olive oil, minced garlic, salt, and pepper. Add water as needed to achieve your desired dressing consistency.

3. **Assemble the Salad:**
   - Drizzle the lemon-tahini dressing over the salad.
   - Toss the salad gently to ensure all ingredients are coated with the dressing.

4. **Serve and Enjoy:**
   - Plate the salad and serve immediately. Enjoy the refreshing and hormone-boosting flavors.

Benefits:
1. **Leafy Greens for Detoxification:**
   - Kale, spinach, and arugula contain chlorophyll and antioxidants, supporting liver detoxification.

2. **Cruciferous Broccoli for Hormonal Balance:**
   - Broccoli contains compounds that may assist in hormone balance.

3. **Cucumber for Hydration:**
   - Cucumber is hydrating and contributes vitamins and minerals essential for overall health.

4. **Pumpkin Seeds for Zinc:**
   - Zinc is important for hormone production, and pumpkin seeds are a good source.

5. **Tahini for Healthy Fats:**
   - Tahini provides healthy fats and adds a creamy texture to the dressing.

Application:

- **Detoxifying Lunch or Dinner:**
  - Enjoy this Hormone-Boosting Detox Salad as a satisfying and detoxifying lunch or dinner option.

- **Regular Detox Routine:**
  - Incorporate this salad into your routine for a period of hormone-boosting and cleansing.

- **Post-Indulgence Reset:**
  - Use this salad as a reset after a period of indulgence or to kickstart a healthier lifestyle.

As with any dietary changes, consult with a healthcare professional or nutritionist for personalized advice, especially if you have specific health concerns or conditions.

Vegetarian Hormone-Supportive Buddha Bowl

Scenario:

Nourish your body and support hormone health with a delicious and nutrient-packed Vegetarian Hormone-Supportive Buddha Bowl.

This recipe incorporates plant-based ingredients rich in essential nutrients to promote hormonal balance. Make this Buddha Bowl a cornerstone of your vegetarian hormone-supportive diet.

Ingredients:

For the Buddha Bowl:

- 1 cup cooked quinoa
- 1 cup chickpeas, roasted with olive oil and spices
- 1 cup broccoli florets, steamed
- 1 cup sweet potato, diced and roasted
- 1/2 avocado, sliced
- 1 cup kale, massaged with olive oil

For the Tahini-Lemon Dressing:

- 2 tablespoons tahini
- Juice of 1 lemon
- 1 tablespoon olive oil
- 1 clove garlic, minced
- Salt and pepper to taste

- Water (as needed to thin the dressing)

Preparation:
1. **Prepare the Buddha Bowl:**
   - In a large bowl or plate, arrange cooked quinoa as the base.

   - Add roasted chickpeas, steamed broccoli florets, roasted sweet potato, sliced avocado, and massaged kale in sections on top of the quinoa.

2. **Make the Tahini-Lemon Dressing:**
   - In a small bowl, whisk together tahini, lemon juice, olive oil, minced garlic, salt, and pepper. Add water as needed to achieve your desired dressing consistency.

3. **Drizzle and Serve:**
   - Drizzle the Tahini-Lemon Dressing over the Buddha Bowl.

4. **Garnish and Enjoy:**
   - Garnish with additional herbs or seeds if desired. Enjoy the Vegetarian Hormone-Supportive Buddha Bowl.

Benefits:
1. **Quinoa's Hormone-Balancing Nutrients:**
   - Quinoa is rich in essential amino acids and contributes to overall hormone balance.

2. **Chickpeas for Plant-Based Protein:**
   - Chickpeas provide protein and fiber, supporting satiety and hormonal health.

3. **Cruciferous Broccoli for Hormone Balance:**
   - Broccoli contains compounds that may assist in hormone balance.

4. **Sweet Potato's Nutrient Density:**
   - Sweet potatoes provide complex carbohydrates, fiber, and essential nutrients.

5. **Avocado's Healthy Fats:**
   - Avocado contributes monounsaturated fats, important for hormone production.

Application:
- **Balanced Lunch or Dinner:**
  - Enjoy this Vegetarian Hormone-Supportive Buddha Bowl as a

satisfying and nutrient-dense lunch or dinner.

- **Regular Hormonal Support:**
  - Make this recipe a regular part of your meal rotation to consistently support hormonal health.

- **Post-Workout Nourishment:**
  - Consume after exercise to replenish energy stores and support hormone balance.

As with any dietary changes, consult with a healthcare professional or nutritionist for personalized advice, especially if you have specific health concerns or conditions.

Keto-Friendly Hormone Reset Chicken and Vegetable Skillet

Scenario:
Embark on a Keto-friendly hormone reset journey with a flavorful and low-carb Chicken and Vegetable Skillet.

This recipe is designed to align with a ketogenic approach while incorporating hormone-supportive ingredients. It's a delicious way to reset your hormones while enjoying a keto-friendly meal.

Ingredients:
For the Chicken and Vegetables:
- 1 pound boneless, skinless chicken thighs, sliced
- 2 tablespoons olive oil
- 1 bell pepper, thinly sliced
- 1 zucchini, spiralized or thinly sliced
- 1 cup cherry tomatoes, halved
- 2 cloves garlic, minced
- 1 teaspoon dried oregano
- Salt and pepper to taste

For the Avocado-Lime Sauce:
- 1 ripe avocado
- Juice of 1 lime

- 2 tablespoons olive oil
- 1 tablespoon fresh cilantro, chopped
- Salt and pepper to taste

Preparation:
1. **Cook the Chicken and Vegetables:**
   - In a large skillet, heat olive oil over medium-high heat.

   - Add sliced chicken thighs and cook until browned on all sides.

   - Add bell pepper, zucchini, cherry tomatoes, minced garlic, dried oregano, salt, and pepper. Sauté until vegetables are tender and chicken is cooked through.

2. **Make the Avocado-Lime Sauce:**
   - In a blender or food processor, combine avocado, lime juice, olive oil, chopped cilantro, salt, and pepper. Blend until smooth.

3. **Combine and Serve:**
   - Pour the Avocado-Lime Sauce over the cooked chicken and vegetables. Toss gently to coat.

4. **Garnish and Enjoy:**
   - Garnish with additional cilantro if desired. Serve the Keto-Friendly Hormone Reset Chicken and Vegetable Skillet immediately.

Benefits:
1. **Chicken for Protein and Healthy Fats:**
   - Chicken thighs provide protein and healthy fats, crucial for hormone production.

2. **Low-Carb Vegetables for Nutrients:**
   - Bell pepper, zucchini, and cherry tomatoes are low-carb and rich in vitamins and minerals.

3. **Avocado's Healthy Fats:**
   - Avocado contributes monounsaturated fats, supporting hormone production and satiety.

4. **Lime for Refreshing Flavor:**
   - Lime adds a zesty and refreshing flavor while providing vitamin C.

Application:
   - **Keto-Friendly Dinner Option:**
     - Enjoy this Chicken and Vegetable Skillet as a satisfying and keto-friendly dinner option.

- **Regular Keto Hormone Reset:**
  - Make this recipe a regular part of your keto hormone-resetting routine to support your low-carb lifestyle.

- **Post-Workout Keto Nourishment:**
  - Consume after exercise to replenish energy stores and support hormone balance while adhering to a ketogenic diet.

As with any dietary changes, consult with a healthcare professional or nutritionist for personalized advice, especially if you have specific health concerns or conditions.

Low-Glycemic Index (GI) Quinoa Salad with Roasted Vegetables

Scenario:

Embrace the benefits of a Low-Glycemic Index (GI) diet with a delicious Quinoa Salad featuring roasted vegetables.

This recipe focuses on incorporating low-GI ingredients to help stabilize blood sugar levels and promote overall well-being. Enjoy this nutritious and satisfying meal as part of your low-GI lifestyle.

Ingredients:

For the Quinoa Salad:

- 1 cup quinoa, rinsed
- 2 cups water
- 1 tablespoon olive oil
- 1 bell pepper (any color), diced
- 1 zucchini, diced
- 1 cup cherry tomatoes, halved
- 1 red onion, thinly sliced
- 2 cloves garlic, minced
- Salt and pepper to taste
- Fresh parsley for garnish

For the Lemon-Tahini Dressing:
- 2 tablespoons tahini
- Juice of 1 lemon
- 2 tablespoons extra-virgin olive oil
- 1 clove garlic, minced
- Salt and pepper to taste
- Water (as needed to thin the dressing)

Preparation:
1. **Cook the Quinoa:**
   - In a saucepan, combine quinoa and water. Bring to a boil, then reduce heat to low, cover, and simmer for 15-20 minutes or until quinoa is cooked. Allow it to cool.

2. **Roast the Vegetables:**
   - Preheat the oven to 400°F (200°C).

   - In a large baking pan, toss diced bell pepper, zucchini, cherry tomatoes, red onion, and minced garlic with olive oil, salt, and pepper.

   - Roast in the oven for 20-25 minutes or until the vegetables are tender and slightly caramelized.

3. **Prepare the Lemon-Tahini Dressing:**
   - In a small bowl, whisk together tahini, lemon juice, olive oil, minced garlic, salt, and pepper. Add water as needed to achieve your desired dressing consistency.

4. **Assemble the Salad:**
   - In a large bowl, combine the cooled quinoa with the roasted vegetables.

   - Drizzle the Lemon-Tahini Dressing over the salad and toss gently to combine.

5. **Garnish and Enjoy:**
   - Garnish with fresh parsley. Serve the Low-Glycemic Index Quinoa Salad at room temperature or chilled.

Benefits:
1. **Low-Glycemic Index Quinoa:**
   - Quinoa has a low glycemic index, providing sustained energy without causing rapid spikes in blood sugar.

2. **Fiber from Vegetables:**
   - Roasted vegetables contribute fiber, aiding in digestion and blood sugar control.

3. **Healthy Fats from Tahini and Olive Oil:**
    - The dressing provides healthy fats, supporting satiety and nutrient absorption.

Application:
- **Balanced Lunch or Dinner:**
    - Enjoy this Low-Glycemic Index Quinoa Salad as a satisfying and balanced lunch or dinner.

- **Regular Low-GI Lifestyle:**
    - Make this recipe a regular part of your low-GI lifestyle to help maintain stable blood sugar levels.

- **Post-Exercise Refuel:**
    - Consume after exercise to replenish energy stores without causing rapid blood sugar spikes.

As with any dietary changes, consult with a healthcare professional or nutritionist for personalized advice, especially if you have specific health concerns or conditions.

Intermittent Fasting Green Protein Smoothie

Scenario:
Embark on your Intermittent Fasting journey with a nutrient-packed Green Protein Smoothie. This recipe is designed to provide essential nutrients while keeping you within the fasting window.

Enjoy this smoothie as part of your intermittent fasting plan, providing a boost of energy and nutrition without compromising your fasting goals.

Ingredients:
For the Green Protein Smoothie:
- 1 cup unsweetened almond milk
- 1 scoop plant-based protein powder
- 1/2 avocado
- 1 cup spinach leaves
- 1/2 cucumber, peeled and sliced
- 1/2 green apple, cored and chopped
- 1 tablespoon chia seeds
- Ice cubes (optional)

For Garnish (optional):
- Sliced almonds or pumpkin seeds
- Fresh mint leaves

Preparation:

1. **Blend the Ingredients:**
   - In a blender, combine almond milk, plant-based protein powder, avocado, spinach, cucumber, apple, and chia seeds.

   - Blend until smooth and creamy. Add ice cubes if a colder consistency is desired.

2. **Pour and Garnish:**
   - Pour the Green Protein Smoothie into a glass.

   - Garnish with sliced almonds or pumpkin seeds for added texture and fresh mint leaves for a burst of flavor.

3. **Enjoy During Fasting Window:**
   - Consume this smoothie during your eating window while practicing intermittent fasting.

Benefits:

1. **Plant-Based Protein:**
   - Plant-based protein powder contributes to muscle maintenance and satiety.

2. **Healthy Fats from Avocado:**
   - Avocado provides monounsaturated fats, aiding in nutrient absorption.

3. **Fiber-Rich Greens:**
   - Spinach and cucumber offer fiber, supporting digestion and a feeling of fullness.

4. **Low-Glycemic Index Apple:**
   - The addition of a green apple provides natural sweetness with a low impact on blood sugar.

Application:
- **Break-the-Fast Option:**
  - Enjoy this Green Protein Smoothie as a nutritious option to break your fast during the eating window.

- **Pre-Workout Fuel:**
  - Consume before a workout for sustained energy and to support muscle function.

- **Morning Boost:**
  - Incorporate into your morning routine for a nutrient-packed start to the day.

Remember, it's crucial to consult with a healthcare professional or nutritionist before beginning any new dietary plan, especially one involving intermittent fasting.

Individual needs and health conditions vary, and personalized advice can ensure you're making choices that align with your specific requirements.

Protein-Packed Paleo Turkey and Vegetable Skewers

Scenario:
Elevate your Paleo journey with these Protein-Packed Turkey and Vegetable Skewers. This recipe focuses on lean proteins and vibrant vegetables, aligning with the principles of the Paleo diet.

Savor the delicious flavors and enjoy the nutritional benefits of a protein-packed Paleo meal.

Ingredients:

For the Turkey Marinade:
- 1.5 pounds turkey breast, cut into cubes
- 2 tablespoons olive oil
- 2 cloves garlic, minced
- 1 teaspoon smoked paprika
- 1 teaspoon ground cumin
- Salt and pepper to taste
- Juice of 1 lemon

For the Vegetable Skewers:
- 1 zucchini, sliced
- 1 bell pepper (any color), diced
- Cherry tomatoes
- Red onion, cut into chunks

- Wooden skewers (soaked in water for 30 minutes)

For Avocado Dipping Sauce:
- 1 ripe avocado
- 2 tablespoons fresh cilantro, chopped
- 1 tablespoon lime juice
- Salt and pepper to taste

Preparation:
1. **Prepare the Turkey Marinade:**
   - In a bowl, combine olive oil, minced garlic, smoked paprika, ground cumin, salt, pepper, and lemon juice.

   - Add turkey cubes to the marinade, ensuring they are well-coated. Let it marinate for at least 30 minutes.

2. **Assemble the Skewers:**
   - Preheat the grill or grill pan.

   - Thread marinated turkey cubes, zucchini slices, bell pepper chunks, cherry tomatoes, and red onion onto the soaked wooden skewers.

3. **Grill the Skewers:**
   - Grill the skewers for 10-15 minutes, turning occasionally, until the turkey is cooked through and vegetables are charred.

4. **Make the Avocado Dipping Sauce:**
   - In a blender, combine ripe avocado, chopped cilantro, lime juice, salt, and pepper. Blend until smooth.

5. **Serve and Enjoy:**
   - Serve the Protein-Packed Paleo Turkey and Vegetable Skewers with the Avocado Dipping Sauce on the side.

Benefits:
1. **Lean Protein from Turkey:**
   - Turkey provides high-quality protein, essential for muscle development and repair.

2. **Colorful Vegetables for Nutrients:**
   - Zucchini, bell pepper, cherry tomatoes, and red onion offer a variety of vitamins and minerals.

3. **Healthy Fats from Avocado:**
   - Avocado contributes monounsaturated fats, supporting overall health and satiety.

Application:
- **Paleo Dinner Delight:**
  - Enjoy these skewers as a satisfying and protein-packed Paleo dinner.

- **Outdoor Grilling Option:**
  - Perfect for summer grilling or any outdoor cooking occasion.

- **Meal Prep Convenience:**
  - Prepare in advance for quick and convenient Paleo meals during the week.

As with any dietary changes, consult with a healthcare professional or nutritionist for personalized advice, especially if you have specific health concerns or conditions.

Hormone-Balancing Berry Green Smoothie

Scenario:

Embark on a Hormone-Balancing Smoothie Cleanse with this refreshing and nutrient-packed Berry Green Smoothie.

Designed to support hormonal balance, this cleanse provides essential vitamins, minerals, and antioxidants. Incorporate this delicious smoothie into your routine to promote overall well-being.

Ingredients:

For the Hormone-Balancing Smoothie:

- 1 cup spinach leaves
- 1/2 cup kale leaves, stems removed
- 1/2 cup blueberries (fresh or frozen)
- 1/2 cup strawberries (fresh or frozen)
- 1/2 banana
- 1 tablespoon flaxseeds
- 1 tablespoon chia seeds
- 1 tablespoon hemp seeds
- 1 cup unsweetened almond milk
- Ice cubes (optional)

Optional Add-Ins:
- 1 tablespoon maca powder (for hormonal support)
- 1/2 avocado (for healthy fats)
- 1 teaspoon bee pollen (as a nutrient boost)

Preparation:

1. **Combine Ingredients:**
   - In a blender, combine spinach, kale, blueberries, strawberries, banana, flaxseeds, chia seeds, hemp seeds, and almond milk.

2. **Optional Add-Ins:**
   - Add maca powder, avocado, or bee pollen if desired for additional hormone-balancing benefits.

3. **Blend Until Smooth:**
   - Blend all ingredients until smooth and creamy. Add ice cubes if you prefer a colder consistency.

4. **Pour and Enjoy:**
   - Pour the Hormone-Balancing Berry Green Smoothie into a glass and savor the delicious, nutrient-packed cleanse.

Benefits:
1. **Leafy Greens for Detoxification:**
   - Spinach and kale contain chlorophyll, aiding in detoxification and hormone balance.

2. **Berries for Antioxidants:**
   - Blueberries and strawberries provide antioxidants, protecting against oxidative stress.

3. **Omega-3 Fatty Acids from Seeds:**
   - Flaxseeds, chia seeds, and hemp seeds contribute omega-3 fatty acids, essential for hormonal health.

4. **Maca Powder for Hormonal Support:**
   - Maca is known for its potential to support hormonal balance.

Application:
- **Morning Hormone Boost:**
   - Start your day with this Hormone-Balancing Smoothie as a nutritious and energizing breakfast.

- **Cleanse Reset:**
   - Use this smoothie as part of a short-term cleanse to reset and rejuvenate your body.

- **Post-Workout Recovery:**
    - Consume after exercise to replenish nutrients and support hormone balance.

As with any dietary changes, consult with a healthcare professional or nutritionist for personalized advice, especially if you have specific health concerns or conditions.

High-Fiber Mediterranean Quinoa Salad

Scenario:

Embark on a journey of health with the High-Fiber Mediterranean Quinoa Salad. Inspired by the Mediterranean diet, this recipe is rich in fiber, nutrients, and flavors that promote well-being.

Incorporate this delicious salad into your routine to enjoy the benefits of a high-fiber Mediterranean lifestyle.

Ingredients:

For the Quinoa Salad:

- 1 cup quinoa, rinsed
- 2 cups water
- 1 cucumber, diced
- 1 cup cherry tomatoes, halved
- 1/2 cup Kalamata olives, pitted and sliced
- 1/2 red onion, finely chopped
- 1/2 cup feta cheese, crumbled
- 1/4 cup fresh parsley, chopped

For the Mediterranean Dressing:

- 1/4 cup extra-virgin olive oil
- 2 tablespoons red wine vinegar
- 1 teaspoon Dijon mustard

- 1 clove garlic, minced
- 1 teaspoon dried oregano
- Salt and pepper to taste

Preparation:
1. **Cook the Quinoa:**
   - In a saucepan, combine quinoa and water. Bring to a boil, then reduce heat to low, cover, and simmer for 15-20 minutes or until quinoa is cooked. Allow it to cool.

2. **Prepare the Salad Ingredients:**
   - In a large bowl, combine the cooked quinoa, diced cucumber, cherry tomatoes, Kalamata olives, chopped red onion, crumbled feta cheese, and chopped fresh parsley.

3. **Make the Mediterranean Dressing:**
   - In a small bowl, whisk together olive oil, red wine vinegar, Dijon mustard, minced garlic, dried oregano, salt, and pepper.

4. **Combine and Toss:**
   - Pour the Mediterranean dressing over the quinoa salad.

- Toss the salad gently to ensure all ingredients are coated with the dressing.

Chill and Serve:
- Refrigerate the salad for at least 30 minutes before serving to enhance the flavors.

- Serve the High-Fiber Mediterranean Quinoa Salad as a refreshing and nourishing meal.

Benefits:
1. **Quinoa for Fiber and Protein:**
   - Quinoa is a complete protein source and a good source of dietary fiber.

2. **Vegetables for Nutrients:**
   - Cucumber, cherry tomatoes, and red onion provide vitamins, minerals, and antioxidants.

3. **Healthy Fats from Olive Oil and Feta:**
   - Extra-virgin olive oil and feta cheese contribute monounsaturated fats, supporting heart health.

4. **Mediterranean Lifestyle Benefits:**
   - This recipe aligns with the Mediterranean diet, known for its

positive effects on heart health and overall well-being.

Application:
- **Lunch or Dinner Option:**
  - Enjoy this High-Fiber Mediterranean Quinoa Salad as a satisfying and nutritious lunch or dinner.

- **Regular Mediterranean Diet:**
  - Make this recipe a regular part of your Mediterranean-inspired meal rotation for long-term health benefits.

- **Meal Prep Convenience:**
  - Prepare in advance for quick and convenient Mediterranean-style meals during the week.

As with any dietary changes, consult with a healthcare professional or nutritionist for personalized advice, especially if you have specific health concerns or conditions.

CONCLUSION

Finally, "The Galveston Diet Book" is your steadfast companion on a transforming path toward long-term weight loss and hormonal balance.

As you finish each chapter, imagine a world in which reaching your health objectives is not only a possibility, but a certainty. This book is the sum of scientific expertise and pragmatism, empowering you to burn fat, easily control hormonal imbalances, and restore your body to its ideal condition.

It's more than a conclusion; it's an invitation to a new world, one in which the complicated dance of hormones becomes a song of well-being and weight reduction becomes a natural expression of balance.

Take the lessons you've learned and the habits you've created and walk boldly into a future where your body and hormones function in harmony, ushering in a life of vigor and joy.

"The Galveston Diet Book" is more than just a conclusion; it heralds a new age in which you have complete control over your health and fitness.

www.ingramcontent.com/pod-product-compliance
Lightning Source LLC
Chambersburg PA
CBHW060959260726
48661CB00005B/1948